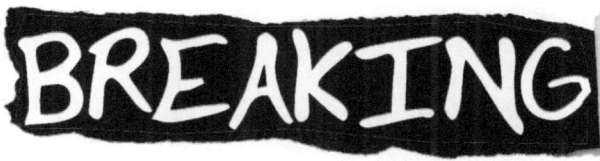

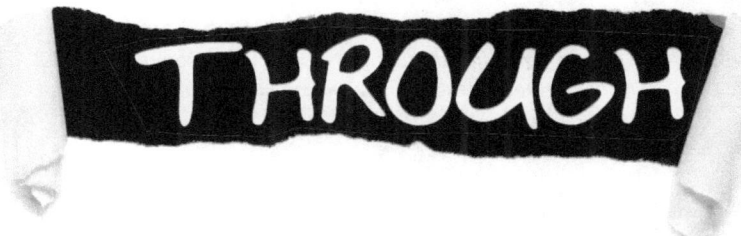

A Common Sense Guide To Losing Weight And Keeping It Off

Theodore H. Valentine

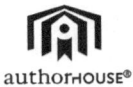

authorHOUSE®

AuthorHouse™
1663 Liberty Drive, Suite 200
Bloomington, IN 47403
www.authorhouse.com
Phone: 1-800-839-8640

First published by AuthorHouse 3/11/2008

ISBN: 978-1-4343-5733-5 (sc)

Library of Congress Control Number: 2008900973

Printed in the United States of America
Bloomington, Indiana

This book is printed on acid-free paper.

Acknowledgments

There are some very special people I would like to thank.

My beautiful wife, Sandie, for your support and belief in me over the years. You have inspired and challenged me to grow to new heights. Alexia Valentine, you were the spark at all the right times. Michelle Traxler, your enthusiasm and excitement on the concepts in the book was contagious. You were a tremendous help in this book getting printed. Steve and Lorraine Brown, your friendship has always been very important to me and it means more to me than you may ever know. You brought new experiences to my life and have made a life long positive impact. Thank you for being the wonderful people that you are. Sandy Mccaslin, Susan Vandenberg and Erika Stell. You have been a tremendous help to me and you are a major influence in my life. I would to thank the all ladies at Preference Mortgage. This is where it all started. From the one page of suggestions I wrote down to help a few of you with your weight loss goals, to your constant request for more information. Kerry Parker and Danette Mitchell, fellow writers and encouragers. Your success as writers and your support over the years has been a great motivation to me.

Brian Mattox, for your e-mails and reminders to get the book finished over the last two years, kept me on track.

7

Contents

ACKNOWLEDGMENTS V

"BREAKING THROUGH" 1

A COMMON SENSE GUIDE TO LOSING WEIGHT AND
KEEPING IT OFF 1

GETTING STARTED 7

FIRST: THE TRUTH ABOUT DIETS 7

THE THREE SIMPLE STEPS .11

    1 – EAT LESS 11

    2 – MOVE MORE 15

    3 – MEAL TIMING 18

EXERCISE SOME CONTROL – IMPLEMENT SOME
CHANGE, AND START BREAKING THROUGH! 23

PART TWO: APPLIED KNOWLEDGE IS POWER 23

STEPS 4 – 5 – 6 – TO SUCCESS 29

    4 – FINDING A PLAN 29

    5 – STAYING CONSISTENT 32

    6 – CREATING TIME 34

LITTLE CHICK 36

WHAT YOU CAN BELIEVE, YOU CAN ACHIEVE! 41

QUICK REFFERENCE GUIDE .41

    1 – EAT LESS 41

    2 – MOVE MORE 43

3 – MEAL TIMING 44

4 – FINDING A PLAN 45

5 – STAYING CONSISTENT 46

6 – CREATING TIME 47

YOU ARE UNIQUE, YOU ARE ONE OF A KIND AND YOU
MATTER! 49

LITTLE CHICK 49

ABOUT THE AUTHOR 53

BREAKING THROUGH

A COMMON SENSE GUIDE
TO LOSING WEIGHT AND KEEPING IT OFF

I would like to thank you for deciding to buy this book. You are going to find that you have made a decision that will affect you for the rest of your life. Just the fact that you are reading this book is telling me that you are at that place in your life, where you are sick-and-tired of being sick-and-tired about your weight and ready to do something about it. Well, I want you to know that you are not alone. There are thousands of people at this very moment feeling just the same as you. The good news is that you can do something about it. There is a plan out there that will work for you; the key is finding a sensible plan that you will work. So, I wrote this book to help you find your plan and to be used as an enhancement to get the best results from your sensible weight loss program. The key word is "sensible". I'll talk about this later on in the book. For now, think of this book as a toolbox full of mental tools; tools that will assist you in losing weight, getting fit and staying that way. This could be one of the most important challenges that some of us will face.

I'll give you some of my personal experiences and the experiences of people who made a positive impact in my life. You will discover different ways of looking at things you may have tried in the past. You will also find yourself saying that the concepts in this book make common sense.

I believe that life is a gift to be cherished and enjoyed. Even though it may seem complicated, it comes down to a series of decisions; good decisions and bad decisions. The good ones we chalk up as great experiences. The bad ones we have to learn to get over. Have you ever made a decision that turned out to be one you wished you hadn't made? Did you find yourself still kicking yourself about it the next day? Or, waking up in the middle of the night tossing and turning saying, "Why did I do that?"

Well, think of it like this. Everyone, at one point or another makes bad decisions. It's getting to the point where you can learn from a bad decision, move forward and not repeat the same bad decisions over and over again. That's what's important. Right?

One of the decisions we make on a constant basis deals with food, what to eat, where to eat, when to eat, how much to eat and so on. Well! Before you start kicking yourself over the shape that you have eaten yourself into, remember that you had a great deal of help getting that way. Think about this. Most of our traditional celebrations are built around eating food. Let's start from the very first day of the New Year, and… how do we celebrate? With a grand dinner and all the trimmings. Right? Don't forget Super Bowl Sunday, how many hot dogs and beer can one person consume? Now what about February? We have Valentine's Day; not only do we fill ourselves up on chocolates, we give it to everyone we know, so they can do the same thing. We take a break in March but start up again in April with Easter. We have a rabbit delivering candy-filled eggs and chocolate bunnies.

We gorge ourselves with food and candy, until we can't stand it. May has Memorial Day; we honor our soldiers, then, make a stop at our favorite restaurant. Hold on to your hats; here comes June and the weather is just right for eating, can you say picnic. Then, BANG! POW! WOW.... It's the 4th of July and .... what's the 4th without barbecue, soda, potato salad, chips, and plenty of sweets. Right?

We do take a break in August, and September would give us a break, except it's Labor Day and we can't be caught laboring in the kitchen, so its picnic time again. Plus, the kids will soon be headed back to school and we squeeze in a vacation and Eat! Eat! Eat! Right? Oh! There'll be no exercising while we're on vacation! Now, it's October and what can I say about October? Hello! Halloween! There's candy and junk food everywhere. We're down to the big two: November and December. There is enough food going into our stomachs during these last two months to feed the entire planet. Hmm, did I forget your birthday and the birthday of everyone you know? Even the restaurants are in on it. If you tell them it's your birthday, you'll get (in some places) free cake and ice cream. Are you getting my point?

You can't take a walk, drive a car, ride a bus, take a train, watch TV, listen to the radio, play a DVD or go online without some type of advertisement about food. Right?

I am sure you will know the answers to these questions:

What will you find at the Golden Arches? – If you want to have it your way, where do you go? – What will you find if you run to the border? – If you want it Hot and Juicy, where do you get it? When you want a Six-Dollar Hamburger for three dollars and ninety-five cents, who will make it for you? How about Pizza! Pizza, do I even need to go there?

So, as you can see, we do have challenges out there. Here's the concern. Food is one of the things that we enjoy in life, and will always be a major part of our celebrations. We have to learn to enjoy it without overdoing it. I know what you are thinking: "If I could do that, I wouldn't be reading this book. Right?" I know. That's why I wrote this book. With a little adjustment to the way we approach weight control, we will achieve our goal. I am not going to tell you that making the decision to lose weight is going to be easy, but I'll tell you this, it will be worth it and I mean every inch!

With all sorts of things going on, I have come to realize that some of the best parts of life are the experiences we create, the experiences we share with others and the positive impact we make on the lives of the people around us. Wouldn't you agree? This book is my way of giving back some of what life has taught me. I know that the challenge with weight control is something that people struggle with every day.

It's also something that could be holding you back from experiencing more of what life has to offer. So, take this tool and apply the principles to your life. Learn to make better decisions. Decide to make good things happen for you.

Make sure you check with your doctor before you start any workout program!

Getting Started

FIRST: THE TRUTH ABOUT DIETS

Diets don't last. This is why. Most diets force you to make unrealistic changes in your eating habits and these unrealistic changes are not easily maintained. Once you stop, you could gain all the weight back, and in most cases, more! There are people who are successful with diets, but most us are not in that elite group. A key would be to find a plan that will work with your lifestyle. Look at eating and exercise as a way to enhance your life. I'll go into more detail later on in the book.

After talking with many people who were successful at losing and maintaining their weight, seeing different diets and reading an assortment of books, I found that there was one common theme that ran through most of them: "**Be sensible**." It's truly a matter of using your common sense.

This hit home with me and was an answer I'd been looking for. If I just use common sense when eating and when exercising, I could lose the weight and, more important, maintain it.

WE DO WHAT WE WANT MOST IN LIFE, NOT WHAT WE WOULD LIKE TO DO IN LIFE:
Neal Askew

There's a big difference between the things we say we would like to do versus the things that we say we want to do. If everyone got what he or she liked in life, we would all be in great physical and mental condition. We would be financially secure, and if we were working, it would be doing something that was meaningful and fulfilling. It would be intellectually challenging and contributing to the betterment of our society. Right? Well, why isn't that the case? It's because the things we say we would like to do are more in line with wishes and wishes don't require effort, discipline or planning. Now, your "wants" are a completely different thing. When you use the word "want", it is normally the step before actually doing something about it. It's more of a decision to discipline yourself, make a plan and do whatever it will take to make what your "wants" a reality.

Example: If I were to say, "I'd **like** to lose 20 pounds". Does it just happen? …..No! Because it's just a nice dream. As though I'll wake up the next day and "poof" the 20 pounds are gone. So, here's the problem.

I **want** to eat cakes, cookies, fried chicken, mashed potatoes and gravy. Does this happen? Yes! …..Because my wanting to eat these things would be the next step before actually doing something about it, which is eating them. Right?

I'd **like** to exercise, but I **want** to lie around watching sports or the soaps on the big screen. You get the point? In this case, I would need to **want** to lose 20 pounds enough to be able to push myself away from the table and the big screen in order to make this a reality. The truth is…. it will be up to you and no one else. I can help you understand some of the hurdles that will be ahead of you. I can also help you understand that with knowledge comes the power to motivate yourself. Yet, it will still ultimately be up to you to make it happen.

THE KEY TO CREATING THE NEW YOU IS CHANGE!

Because we do what we <u>want</u> most, we must <u>want</u> to change our eating habits. I'll be the first one to tell you that it is not an easy thing to do; however, it can be done. You just have to give yourself enough time and understand how your body works. That's why diets don't last. Your mind, unfortunately, needs more time to accept the changes you're required to make with some diets. So, your mind rejects the plan and you have to force yourself to keep it going. Soon your **wants** win you over and you **want** to stop the diet. Right?

Here's the skinny (no pun intended), you didn't put on the weight overnight and you are not going to lose it overnight. So, be kind to yourself and remember this is going to be a journey. I know using the word journey makes it sound as though it will be fun. Well, that's just what I want it to sound like. If I can make it fun for you, or at least enjoyable, you'll keep doing it.

The Three Simple Steps

1 – EAT LESS
MOVE MORE –
MEAL TIMING

---
1 – EAT LESS

It's well known that if you eat more food than your body needs for energy, it will store as fat cells for later use; however, when you need to create more energy you eat again and never use the fat cells your body had stored from the last meal. There's the first of our problems. Most of us eat way too much. Then there are some of us that are going in the opposite direction; after gaining extra weight, you try not eating anything at all. All this does is throw your body into a starvation mode. Your body thinks that it will not get more food. So, it holds on to every fat cell it can and slows down your metabolism. I know you've heard people say, "I don't eat very much and I am not losing weight." Right?

It's very likely this is going on in their life. Everything in life needs balance, including the food you eat. There are many books out there that can help you find the right balance of food that is best for you. Here are some things that will help you:

- Don't make radical changes in your eating habits at first– cut back on the amount that you are currently eating. If you are eating two servings of food, cut it back to one.

  If you are eating two burgers, make it one. You know what I am talking about. When you see the changes in the way you look and associate the changes with your new plan, you will **want** to make healthier choices.

- Choose alternatives – you could have a glass of water, a salad or an orange/apple before your main meal. This will make it easier to put less on your plate. Cut back on the amount of soda you are drinking. You will be surprised at the changes you will see by cutting down on sodas. You don't have to stop drinking soda altogether, just not every day.

  I ran into a friend that I had not seen in a while. She was a few sizes smaller and I asked her what she was doing to lose the weight. She told me that she started walking in the evenings and replaced the sodas she was drinking with water. She lost 15 pounds. Do you think this is going to help her stay motivated? You bet it will!

- Understand that you are used to eating a certain amount of food. When you eat less, you may feel hungry, but it's more likely that you're just used to that familiar amount food and now you are doing something different. If you wait about 10-20 minutes, you'll feel satisfied, not full. You don't want to have that stuffed full feeling anymore.

That stuffed feeling is a sign that you are overeating. If you don't feel quite satisfied, eating a little more will do the job.

- When you are going out for dinner, don't be afraid to ask for your salad or soup prior to ordering your main meal. This will help you choose your main course more wisely.

You don't want to order your food on an empty stomach.

You may find that your soup/salad was just the right amount and now you're ready for the good stuff, a small main dish and maybe a light dessert. This will help you. Restaurants are in the business to please their customers. They will do whatever they can to ensure that you have a great dining experience. The restaurant owner's goal is to have you return with family and friends and recommend their restaurant. With this knowledge, you now have the power to take control and make your dining out experience more pleasurable.

- If you are like most people, once food is on your plate, it's hard not to eat it. So, ask your server to take it off before you get it. Some restaurants have half orders and, if not, you can ask for a smaller serving. You'll feel better about your night out and, if you're happy, the owner is happy.

Do you remember a few years back when people would say they were on a "see food diet"? They see food and they eat it! Well, this is the reverse; we don't see food, so we don't eat it!

• Learn to become sensitive to what your body is telling you. You'll find that different foods will cause you to have a wide variety of feelings. For instance, I have to be aware of the amount of milk I drink. Don't get me wrong; I enjoy milk but, if I drink too much, I feel bloated and not very energetic. So, I've had to cut back on the amount I drink everyday.

You could find that some foods you eat will give you energy and some foods you eat will make you feel absolutely lousy. These are the types of things you need to know about yourself, because how you feel will determine the amount of effort that you will put forth in order to be successful.

2 – MOVE MORE

You can make this area fun, because there are so many ways that you could find to move more. The trick will be to find something that you are going to like and stick with.

The best way to determine this will be to get out there and try some different things. Believe me, I know that in the past you may not have wanted to do anything. But, today's a new day and you are a new person and remember, attitude is everything and you have to learn to keep it in check. Try calling some of your friends and join them in some of the things they enjoy doing. If you don't have friends, this will be a good time to make some. When you get out in the active world, you are going to meet other people that like the things that you are trying and you'll have something in common built in.

My wife recently joined a mountain bike club in our town called "RATS" (Rockville Alternative Transportation System) and the "Bike Me" road cycling club. By joining the clubs, she has brought an entirely new group of people into her life, all with their own experiences and other interests, things that my wife may not have thought of doing. You wouldn't believe some of the stories I have heard. So! Have some fun with this; get out there and try new things.

Here are some ideas that will help you:

- Be careful about making radical changes right away – here is an example: If you haven't been to the gym in ages you may not want to start an everyday routine. You could become very sore and discouraged. I think you know what comes next: **"I quit!"**

Start by doing a little more than you were doing in the past. That could be an easy thing, if you weren't doing anything at all. The main thing is to have "fun."

- You could start out by walking around your block or going a few days a week to the gym and using the treadmill. Remember, only you know where you are now and what you **have or haven't** been doing in the past. Don't let other people intimidate you and persuade you to push yourself too hard in the beginning.

Sometimes people forget where they started. They forget when they couldn't make it through the entire step-class or even run around the block without stopping. By starting off easy, you can give yourself a chance to find pleasure in your new workout.

Remember, it took time to put on the extra weight and it will take time to work it off!

- Try doing some type of exercise before you go to bed – it will get your metabolism working for you overnight. It doesn't have to be anything fancy. That's all going to depend on your current physical condition and how much you want to do!

- It could be that you are going to do some jumping jacks, push-ups, and crunches. Maybe you have a treadmill and you spend some time on that. It could be that you are going to the gym in the evening, first thing in the morning or in the afternoon. I have a friend that has a flexible work schedule and he's able to go to the gym at lunch. You get the point. Make something work for you. **That's the important thing.**

- Here is the main point about moving more: You have to learn to burn more calories than you take in. That may sound simple but that's just the way it's. This is the main key to weight control. **Move to burn more calories than you eat!**

3 – MEAL TIMING

It's just as important <u>when</u> you eat as <u>what</u> you eat, if not more important.

I remember there was a time in my life when my friends were saying, "Theo, you look good. What have you been doing?" I was still eating the same types and amount of food. The only thing I had changed was not eating so late at night. I ate my dinner earlier in the evening and had some fruit or something light if I felt the need for something more.

- Be aware that there are certain foods that you can eat in the morning and you can't or shouldn't eat at night. For example: I like to eat cold fried chicken and if I eat it in the morning I am fine, however, if I have it at night, it feels like I have a rock in my stomach. It's the same way with milk. I can drink it in the morning but I stay away from it at night. Recognizing how you feel after the foods you eat will become more important as you move along through this program.

- Leave some time between when you eat and when you sleep. Leave about 3 hours between the time you eat a heavy meal and go to sleep. I know this won't always be possible. With a busy lifestyle you may not have three hours before you sleep. So, you will have to be creative. There are times when I just eat an apple instead of what I had planned to eat. I needed to get to bed. In the morning I was glad I ate less.

Remember, what your body doesn't use, it stores as fat cells.

You don't want that!

- Try to have your heavy meals earlier in the day. Try having a more satisfying lunch and a lighter dinner. You have to find what works better for you. We are not all the same and it's very important to remember that! As you become more aware of this, you will begin making faster progress.

- Be sensible, don't over do it on the **fatty stuff.** You can still have the things you like, *just don't over do it!* Start reminding yourself of what you are trying to achieve. It will help you maintain control over how much and what you eat. You'll surprise yourself. Once you start having this kind of control in your life, you will be amazed at what you can achieve!

- Have a small slice of cake, **not a chunk of cake!** Do you really need to eat the entire stack of pancakes, two strips of bacon and two sausages? Just because you can buy it doesn't mean you have to eat it. How about the 48-ounce soda, jumbo dog and stuffing yourself at the all-you-can-eat buffets? Is a triple cheeseburger with double bacon on a sesame seed bun, something that you truly ought to buy? No; and just because you add avocado, lettuce and tomato, doesn't make it a healthy meal either. Also, after eating all that food, you know you're not going to feel good! Plus, if you ate all that the next thing you would be saying would be "I can't believe I ate that, it feels like there is a rock in my stomach, I feel bloated" you know the story. There are companies that have made a fortune off of us feeling that way. Do you remember the commercial that went "Plop- Plop-Fizz-Fizz, Oh what a relief it is"? You drop two of these tablets into a glass of water when you have over-eaten and have that bloated feeling. They have made millions if not billions of dollars from us eating until we feel just miserable.

- There may be times when you have to talk to yourself, if that's what it takes to get back under control. One day, Erika, one of my co-workers, was telling me that she was going to take her exercising to the next level. Now, what you need to know about Erika is that she already looks fantastic. Well, around Christmas, it seemed to me that Erika was having a little sweet binge. She was just about to eat something and stopped. I overheard her say very softly, "Erika, Stop It!" She put down what she was going to eat and went back to working on her project. I thought to myself, how awesome. Sometimes, you do whatever it takes if you find yourself doing something that will take you away from your goal.

Here's something else that helped me during those times when I had a weak moment. I heard this in an empowering management class, taught by a lady by the name of Randy Martin.

"Don't let your mood determine your actions.

Stay true to your commitments and your mood will follow."

This is very true and extremely powerful, because your moods are not always going to line up with what you are working to achieve.

Example:

Have you ever planned to do something and when the time came, you didn't feel like doing it? You weren't in a very good mood, but you decided to do it anyway or someone else convinced you. After the event was over, you found that you had a good time and were glad that you did it? That's why this is so important.

There has been times when I have come home and my wife would say "lets go for a walk" and here is the truth; I really didn't feel like going for the walk, but I did want to be with her so, I went. And I'll tell you, there hasn't been one time when I went, even though I didn't feel like it, that after waking I didn't turn to my wife and say that I was glad that she asked me to go. I felt better, had new found energy and a more exciting evening. So, every time you get in one of those, "I don't feel like it moods," remind yourself of that statement and it will encourage you to stick to what you have committed to. You'll find that this will help you in almost every situation. I ran into Sandy, a friend of mine from the banking industry, and Sandy had the statement hanging on the wall in her office. We were discussing different things that we use to keep motivated. She reminded me of our class, and how that statement was helpful to her and her husband as they built their real estate business.

Exercise Some Control - Implement Some Change, and start Breaking Through!

Part one of the book was created to help you make a few mental and physical adjustments. Also, to motivate you to achieve visual success so that you would feel empowered and in control of your new direction in life. This may be the first real physical success you are able to maintain over the long term. My plan for you is to see the changes in your body and feel the difference in your clothes; the old clothes that used to ride up in the wrong places and had those odd puffs. Not a pretty sight. When you see and feel the difference, you'll want to keep going. When you feel that difference, it will make you want to scream to top of your lungs **"YES!"** That's what I am talking about.

When I first started talking to people about this subject, I used to say to my friends "Knowledge is power." But over the years, I've come to realize that's not necessarily accurate. The fact that you know where to get the knowledge or that you even have the knowledge, doesn't really matter, unless you decide to use it. For example: You want to learn to operate a computer. You could go out and buy a book, take it home and place it on your nightstand. So, now you know where to find the knowledge. You could even sit down and read it.

Now you have the knowledge; however, it's not until you actually turn on the computer and apply your new acquired knowledge that you will fulfill your goal. Right?

It's the same thing with your wanting to lose weight and maintain it. You will not see progress until you start applying the principles that you are learning from this book to your life. Just having the knowledge or knowing where to get the knowledge is not going to move you in the right direction. That is why I had to change from saying knowledge is power, to "Applied Knowledge is Power." Doesn't that make more sense?

Congratulations!

Now that you have gotten this far, you are ready to create the "want" in "**We do what we want most in life.**" As we get more into it, there will be three new steps that you'll need to understand in order to reach your new goal. I know, I said the bad five-letter word "GOALS" but remember, you have a whole new outlook on your body and change. Plus! Goals are only a problem when you don't understand how to use them and you find yourself setting unrealistic ones. Like I am going to lose thirty-five pounds in three days and fit in the pants I wore when I was sixteen. These types of goals set you up for failure and we are not going to have any of those here. Right?

Here's something that will help you keep on track. It takes about six weeks of doing something different in order to change a bad habit or to create a new one. Remember what I said earlier in the book, we are all different; so it may take you a little more or less time. The point is that it will take being consistent before it will come naturally to you.

Sometimes it feels as though you have to trick your own body in order to make the gains that you are seeking. We all know that being overweight is unhealthy, yet your body becomes used to the way you are; and it is that familiar feeling that makes it difficult to move forward in your goal to lose weight.

Let's take increasing your strength, for instance. It would be nice if you could work out with heavier weights one day, and the next day be stronger. Right? But, that is not the way it works. The reality would be that you become sore the next day, as though your body was saying, "I didn't like that, so cut it out." If you give in to that feeling, you won't increase your strength at all; however, if you continue to work out, even though you may not feel like it, your strength will increase. It would be as though your body is now saying, "OK, I don't like this, but if you're going to keep this up I am going to get stronger so that this increased weight doesn't cause me pain."

The muscle grows and all you have to do is keep repeating this process. It's the same with losing weight; your body doesn't want that uncomfortable feeling, so it attempts to keep you in your comfort zone.

My friend, Toni, was telling me one day that she had knee surgery about a year ago. She was laid up for some time and had picked up a few extra pounds. Her doctor told her that she should lose some weight, advised her to cut back on the food she was eating and buy a stationary bike to ride at home. (I like this doctor already.) She said after a few weeks she stepped on a scale and, to her surprise, she had gained six pounds. So, she called her doctor and told him that she will not be riding any more.

This is the type of story that I hear too often, because there isn't enough information available that is written in a straight, no hype layperson language.

The problem would be, when you start doing different things to lose weight there are a variety of obstacles that could lead you astray. Mainly, false signs of progress that, in the beginning, could discourage you. One of these obstacles would be the fact that muscle weighs more than fat, so it's possible to stay at the same weight or even gain weight, yet be one or two dress/pants sizes smaller.

Another one of those obstacles could be retaining water because of the high sodium content in the food we eat. You could be moving along losing weight but due to the high sodium content in the food you ate, hold on to the excess water in your body. Jump on the scale and be disappointed and discouraged to find that you are the same weight you were before you started working out or worse, beyond that point.

This could have happened to you in the past and led you to say, "Why work out this hard just to gain all the weight right back." That's why it's so important that you use your clothes and the mirror as your guide in the beginning and stay away from the scale. Repeat after me. "The scale is not your friend." After you are comfortable with how your body is working the scale will not be discouraging.

The next three steps will show you how to choose a plan, why it's important to stay consistent and a way to make time your friend. Enough said! Now let's get to work. Oops! I did it again. Correction, let's get started.

STEPS 4 – 5 – 6 – TO SUCCESS

4 – FINDING A PLAN
STAYING CONSISTENT –
CREATING TIME

4 – FINDING A PLAN

There are more plans available to help you lose weight than there are casinos in Las Vegas. Your challenge will be to find a sensible plan that will work for you and that you will work. I believe any sensible plan will work. Would you like to know why? **"When the student is ready, the teacher appears."** This just means that when you are truly ready and have decided to do something important, you look at life from a different point of view. You find words of wisdom and things of value in places you had not looked before. I believe it's because you are looking for positive things in life that will help you achieve your goals. The tough part will be getting yourself to the point where you **want** to make the changes, not the plan you choose.

- Find a plan that is reasonable for you. You know better than anyone else what you are willing to commit to and also what is not realistic for you.

- You can join a gym, an athletic club, or an organized program like Weight Watchers or Jenny Craig. You could work out at home. There are great books, videos, and personal trainers available. With videos you could go from Tae Bo (Billy Blank) to Richard Simmons. These two guys are radically different, yet they are both extremely effective.

  My family likes the Tae Bo video. We are not that good at it, but the main thing is that we are having fun. You have to learn to enjoy the things that will lead you to your goals. Try walking, jogging or running. This may seem odd, but have you ever seen an overweight sprinter? There must be something to that!

- You could try yoga, walking or cycling. I started road riding and mountain biking and between the two of them I am having fun, as well as controlling my weight.

- You have to be truthful with yourself. You have most likely heard the saying, "You can fool most of the people some of the time and some of the people most of the time, but you can't fool yourself." You know when you are really trying and when you are not! If you're not the type that does well working out alone, you need to join a gym, hire a personal trainer or find a friend to work out with you.

The benefit of a personal trainer or training partner is that you have someone to hold you accountable. If you are the type that does well on your own, any option will work for you. The point here is, if you are not going to put in the effort that is needed, do not expect to see the results you want.

You will need a combination of aerobic exercise and strength training. Some people believe that all they need to do is work out with weights (strength training) and some people believe that all they need is aerobic exercise, and it will get them to their goal. Well, they're half-right! You need both: your aerobic to burn off that fat, love handles, thunder thighs, jelly belly (you know all the terms), and strength training to firm up your arms, legs, thighs, chest and buns.

This is why your program has to have a balance of both aerobic exercise and strength training.

5 – STAYING CONSISTENT

This is very important to your success. Being consistent is not the easiest thing to do, but it's probably the most important.

You'll find it very difficult to make the changes in your body without being consistent in your plan. This is where most people blow it. I think we can all identify with this. You have everything lined up, all your ducks are in a row and then the obstacles start getting in the way. You have to get creative and get around those obstacles.

- It takes about six weeks of doing something to make a new habit or to break an old one. Right? Well, it will take being consistent with your new workout program so it can become a great new habit and one you will stick with.

- Decide how many days you will work your program. Again be realistic! (Remember that an unrealistic goal leads to failure.) It's OK to start with only a few days of working out and staying consistent versus setting up too many days and not being able to stick with it. You will increase your workout when the time is right. I have faith in you!

- Pick a time that will work for you. If you are doing one of the at-home programs, it could be fairly easy; however, you'll have to keep all distractions from interrupting your workout. This could be very challenging but achievable.

If you are using a gym/club, they do offer twenty-four hour clubs and most gym/clubs open very early and close fairly late, just to provide the convenience for you to be consistent. Remember no excuses! Here's something that my friend, Sandy, always says,

"Excuses are Useless."

6 – CREATING TIME

We all know that you cannot create time; however, we all have the same twenty-four hours in a day and it's what we do with our twenty-four hours that's going to make the difference in what we accomplish in life. It's too easy to say, "I don't have time." That is something we hear too often. Right? But is that really true? Think about this. If you got a call from the State Lotto and the person said you won, come down and pick up your money. Would you say, "I don't have time?" No, you would make the time to pick up the money. Right?

Well, aren't we talking about your life? **Isn't your life as important?**

- You have to create the time in your day to make the changes that you want. It may seem difficult, but it only takes making a decision. I know it's not going to be easy, and I also know that you are very busy, but think about this. I am only talking about an hour a day and, as busy as you are, don't you deserve to take one hour out of your day to improve your health for the rest of your life?

- If you have a tight work or school schedule, you will have to become better at planning your workout schedule. It may seem impossible, but it's not. When you are ready to do something, you'll make the time!

- You have to give yourself time to see the change in your body. Other people may see it before you do. **Don't get discouraged**. You see yourself every day and change is gradual, it's harder for you to recognize it, just understand that it's happening!

Now, we are back to, "It takes about six weeks of doing something to make a new habit or to break an old one." It also works with making changes in your body. It takes about six weeks of being consistent with your program before you'll start seeing real change. Now that you know this, don't get discouraged after a few weeks.

This is where most people quit, and feel they have wasted their time. They're wrong! Had they just stuck with it a little longer they would have made it.

"Don't fall for this trick"

- There may be times where you will blow it! Remember we are human and not perfect. If you blow it, don't give up and start saying things like: I knew it, I never stick with anything, I'll never change, etc. You know what I am talking about! Dust yourself off and say, "I blew it,

... it's not the end of the world. I'll just start back on my plan." Remember Nike's words, **"Just Do It."** You're further along than you think you are!

• Now that you have this new (for some of you reconfirmed) knowledge, it's time to apply it to your life. One of the best things you could do would be to go back, revisit the book, and highlight the strategies. As you start developing your new habits, the principles will take on new meaning, plus it can help you stay motivated.

"Nothing Good Comes From Being Overweight"

You are unique, You are one of a kind and You matter!

Here is something to encourage you. When I was in the financial services industry, I heard this story of the "Eagle and the Chicken" told in many different ways, by different people. A gentleman named Neal Askew told the version that made the greatest impact on me. Here is my version:

LITTLE CHICK

Once upon a time, not too long ago, in a place not too far from where you live, was the nest of an eagle. It was on the side of a cliff near the mountains top, and at the base of the cliff was the nest of Mother Prairie Chicken, who spent most of her time in the nest or running around the prairie scratching and digging for worms to eat.

One day while the eagle was away, one of the eggs fell out of the nest and rolled down the mountain into the prairie chicken's nest. After some time had passed, the eggs hatched. Mother Prairie Chicken noticed that one of her chicks was larger than the rest, so she named it Little Chick. Early one morning while Mother Prairie Chicken was teaching her chicks how to scratch and dig for worms, Little Chick looked up and saw this beautiful bird with her enormous wings spread, soaring through the air as if she were dancing on a cloud. Little Chick said "Mommy, mommy, what's that?"

"That's an eagle, the most prestigious of all the birds," said Mother Prairie Chicken. "What is it doing?" Uttered Little Chick. "She's flying, Little Chick," expressed Mother Prairie Chicken. Little Chick shouted, "Can I do that, can I do that?" "No! Little Chick, we are prairie chickens and prairie chickens don't fly. Eagles fly, now go back to scratching and digging for worms," Mother Prairie Chicken said.

The very next day Little Chick was out looking for the eagle. After a few minutes, Little Chick saw the eagle, but this time she was diving toward the still blue waters of this magnificent lake. She scooped something out of the water and was soaring back up to the mountaintop. "Mommy, mommy what was that?" Said Little Chick.

Mother Prairie Chicken said, "That was a fish. Eagles eat fish!" Little Chick's stomach was growling by now, she never could eat enough worms to fill her tummy. Little Chick said, "Mommy, mommy, can we eat fish?" Mother Prairie Chicken expounded, "No! We don't eat fish. We are prairie chickens, we don't fly, we don't eat fish, and we don't live high on the mountaintops. We scratch and dig for worms and run around the prairie."

There may be people in your life telling you that you are a prairie chicken. That you have always been overweight; you're trying another diet; weren't you supposed to have lost 30 pounds last week; you may as well just forget about it, you can't do that; where are you going to find the time; you're not overweight you just have big bones. These people may have the best intentions. They just don't understand that anything you want to accomplish will require some type of risk.

They may think they are keeping you from getting hurt but never-the-less, it's still like Mother Prairie Chicken. All Little Chick needed was someone to believe in her and to say, "You can do this, I believe in you Little Chick." What do you think would have happened with little Chick?

Sometimes all we need to get started is to have someone to believe in us in the beginning stages, before we build the strength to believe in ourselves. I see you as an eagle and I believe with all of my heart that if you want this, it will happen for you.

By the way, remember Little Chick? One day when she was at the edge of the lake watching the eagles soar, one of the eagles seemed to be flying toward Little Chick. Little Chick didn't know what to do, she couldn't move.

The eagle landed right in front of Little Chick and the eagle was even more beautiful than Little Chick could have ever imagined. The Eagle looked down at Little Chick and with tears in her eyes said, "I knew I would find you. I never stopped believing that one day we would be together again." Little Chick couldn't say a word and, in the smallest voice, she said, "Me, are you talking about me? I am Little Chick, the Prairie Chicken, not an eagle." "No Little Chick, you're an eagle and you're my daughter that I have never stopped loving. You were so active in your shell that one day you rolled out of my nest, down the mountain and was thought never to be seen again."

The eagle continued, "It seemed that every day when I flew over the lake I felt as though you were with me and now you are. Let's go home." Little Chick said, "You mean I can......" "Yes! Little Chick, you can fly."

Little Chick spread her enormous wings and with one flap she soared high above the mountaintop.

What You Can Believe, You Can Achieve!

QUICK REFFERENCE GUIDE

---
1 – EAT LESS

- Don't make radical changes in your eating habits at first – cut back on the amount that you are currently eating.

- Choose alternatives – you could have a glass of water, a salad or an orange/apple before your main meal.

Understand that you are used to eating a certain amount of food. When you eat less, you may feel hungry, but it's more likely that you're just used to that familiar amount of food and now you are doing something different.

- When you are going out for dinner, don't be afraid to ask for your salad or soup prior to ordering your main meal.

- Restaurants are in the business to please their customers. They will do whatever they can to ensure that you have a great dining experience.

- Learn to become sensitive to what your body is telling you.

  You could find that some foods you eat will give you energy and some foods you eat will make you feel absolutely lousy.

2 – MOVE MORE

- You could start out by walking around your block or going a few days a week to the gym and using the treadmill.

- Try doing some type of exercise before you go to bed – it will get your metabolism working for you overnight.

Here is the main point about moving more: You have to learn to burn more calories than you take in. That may sound simple but that's just the way it's. This is the main key to weight control. <u>Move to burn more calories than you eat!</u>

3 – MEAL TIMING

- Be aware that there are certain foods that you can eat in the morning and you can't or shouldn't eat at night.

- Leave some time between when you eat and when you sleep.

  Remember, <u>what your body doesn't use, it stores as fat cells.</u> ***You don't want that!***

- Try to have your heavy meals earlier in the day.

- Be sensible, don't over do it on the **fatty stuff.** You can still have the things you like, ***just don't over do it!*** Start reminding yourself of what you are trying to achieve.

- There may be times when you have to talk to yourself, if that's what it takes to get back under control.

4 – FINDING A PLAN

- Find a plan that is reasonable for you. You know better than anyone else what you are willing to commit to and what is not realistic for you.

- You can join a gym, an athletic club, an organized program (like Weight Watchers, Jenny Craig, etc.) or work out at home. There are great books, videos, and personal trainers available.

- You have to be truthful with yourself. You can fool most of the people some of the time and some of the people most of the time, but you can't fool yourself. The point here is, if you are not going to put in the effort that is needed, do not expect to see the results you want.

- You will need a combination of aerobic exercise and strength training. You need both: your aerobics to burn off the fat, love handles, thunder thighs jelly belly (you know all the terms), and strength training to firm up your arms, legs, thighs, chest and buns.

5 – STAYING CONSISTENT

- It takes about six weeks of doing something to make a new habit or to break an old one. It will take being consistent with your new workout program so it can become a great new habit and one you will stick to.

- Decide how many days you will work your program. Again be realistic! (Remember that an unrealistic goal leads to failure.) It's OK to start with only a few days of working out and staying consistent versus setting up too many days and not being able to stick with it.

- Pick a time that will work for you. If you are doing one of the at-home programs, it could be fairly easy; however, you'll have to keep all distractions from interrupting your workout. If you are using a gym/club, they do offer twenty-four hour clubs and most gym/clubs open very early and close fairly late, just to provide the convenience for you to be consistent.

"Excuses are Useless."

6 – CREATING TIME

- You have to create the time in your day to make the changes that you want. It may seem difficult, but it only takes making a decision. I am only talking about an hour a day. Don't you deserve to take one hour out of your day to improve your health for the rest of your life?

- If you have a tight work or school schedule, you will have to become better at planning your workout schedule.

- You have to give yourself time to see the change in your body.

    Don't get discouraged. You see yourself every day and change is gradual, it's harder for you to recognize it, just understand that it's happening!

- There may be times where you will blow it!   Remember we are human and not perfect. Dust yourself off and say, "I blew it, it's not the end of the world. I'll just start back on my plan. Remember, you're further along than you think.

You are unique, You are one of a kind and You matter!

LITTLE CHICK

There may be people in your life telling you that you are a prairie chicken. That you have always been overweight; you're trying another diet; weren't you supposed to have lost 30 pounds last week; you may as well just forget about it, you can't do that; where are you going to find the time; you're not overweight you just have big bones. These people may have the best intentions. They just don't understand that anything you want to accomplish will require some type of risk.

They may think they are keeping you from getting hurt but never-the-less, it's still like Mother Prairie Chicken. All Little Chick needed was someone to believe in her and to say, "You can do this, I believe in you Little Chick." What do you think would have happened with little Chick?

Sometimes all we need to get started is to have someone to believe in us in the beginning stages, before we build the strength to believe in ourselves.

49

I see you as an eagle and I believe with all of my heart that if you want this, it will happen for you.

"WHAT YOU EXPECT TO ACHIEVE, YOU MUST FIRST BELIEVE"

Theodore H. Valentine

About the Author

Theodore H. Valentine, in addition to being a musician, is an avid road cyclist, mountain bicyclist and skilled in the martial arts. Along with Steve Brown former trainer and owner of Astro's Gym, assisted in training and designing the routines for Sandie Valentine's successful winnings of Miss Western America, Miss Michael Angelo and Miss California (Short Class) body building competition in the 80's. His life's passion is helping people do better in life, and now lives in Northern California with wife and three daughters, Krystal, Alexia and Malina.